THE MEDITERRANEAN DIET:

The Complete Guide to Losing Weight and Reducing Your Risk of Heart Disease

By

JAMES H. KINGSLEY

INTRODUCTION

Nowadays, when we think of a "diet," we often think of some kind of restriction that would help us reach a certain objective, like weight loss. The Mediterranean diet does not function in any way like that. Instead, it encourages a dietary pattern that includes foods popular among people who live in the Mediterranean region.

Additionally, it emphasizes the social side of eating, such as getting together with loved ones and having enjoyable conversations over meals.

You'll learn that Mediterranean dieters place a high priority on a plant-based diet that is rich in vegetables and includes good fats like olive oil and omega-3 fatty acids from fish in their meals. It is a diet with a strong track record for heart health.

This diet consists primarily of whole grains and is supplemented with olive oil, fish, nuts, legumes, fruits, and vegetables. If you wish to follow this diet, then you must limit or completely avoid dairy products, sweets, and red meat (though small amounts like yogurt and cheese are included).

If you stick to this diet, you won't have room on your plate for processed foods. Standard cuisine like chicken could be more of a side dish than vegetables, which is what people would notice first when they look at a platter, and it should be colorful.

One feature that many people like about the Mediterranean diet is that it allows for small to moderate amounts of red wine. The recommended daily maximum for "moderate" consumption is 5 ounces (Oz), or around one glass. It's crucial to remember that this eating plan does not mandate that you drink one glass of wine every day, and if you don't already, this restriction does not constitute a suggestion that you start.

Chapter one

What exactly does a Mediterranean diet entail?

There are numerous definitions for the term "diet" (each with slightly different goals for servings). This is so because the diet emphasizes common eating behaviors more than precise math or algorithms. Additionally, it considers the variety of culinary customs followed in Mediterranean countries, each of which has its own distinctive features. Due to its lack of a rigid definition, the Mediterranean diet is flexible and may be adapted to your individual needs.

The term "Mediterranean diet" describes a wide range of eating habits that are popular in countries that are adjacent to the Mediterranean Sea. No specific Mediterranean diet is regarded as the standard. There are at least 16 countries that encircle the Mediterranean. Due to variances in culture, ethnic background, religion, economy, geography, and agricultural output, these countries and even specific regions within each of them have different eating habits. There are, however, a few commonalities.

You'll often consume a lot of vegetables, fruit, beans, lentils, and nuts if you stick to a Mediterranean diet.

- An abundance of healthful grains, like brown rice and whole-wheat bread.

- A lot of EVOO (extra virgin olive oil), which is a good source of healthy fat.

- Moderate amounts of fish, particularly those omega-3-rich fish.

- Some yogurt and cheese, but not too much.

- Choosing chicken over red meat and eating little to no meat.

- Few or no sweets, sugary beverages, or butter.

• Moderate wine consumption with meals (but avoid starting to drink if you don't already).

A nutritionist can help you make any adjustments to this diet that may be required based on your medical history, underlying issues, food preferences, and food allergies.

What benefits does following a Mediterranean diet provide?

One benefit of the Mediterranean diet is that your risk of cardiovascular disease is decreased.

• Sustaining a healthy body weight.

• Helping to keep blood pressure, blood sugar, and cholesterol levels within normal ranges.

• Reducing the likelihood that metabolic syndrome will develop.

• Promoting the maintenance of a healthy balance in the gut microbiota, which is composed of bacteria and other microorganisms and is found in your digestive system.

• Lower chance of contracting particular malignancies.

• Postponing cognitive decline brought on by aging.

• encouraging a longer life expectancy.

The Mediterranean diet is frequently suggested by cardiologists because of the vast research that demonstrates its heart-healthy advantages. In one trial, participants at high risk of cardiovascular disease were followed for five years. Two groupings of these individuals were formed. One group followed a low-fat diet, while the other followed the Mediterranean diet. Comparing the Mediterranean Diet group to the low-fat diet group, cardiovascular events were 30% less likely in the Mediterranean Diet group. These occurrences included heart attacks, strokes, or deaths from cardiovascular causes.

Researchers think that the healthy fats you consume as part of the Mediterranean diet contribute to these protective advantages. Foods including fish, almonds, and olive oil are sources of these.

Chapter two

What unique advantages does the Mediterranean diet offer us?

The diverse nutrients found in the Mediterranean diet help your body in various ways, each in a unique way. None of the benefits of the Mediterranean diet can be linked to just one part or component. The diet is good for your health because it offers a balanced diet.

Take into account a group of several vocalists, like a chorus. The song's full impact can only be achieved when all the voices are heard, even though one vocal might be able to carry some of the melodies on its own. Similarly, the Mediterranean diet boosts your health by providing you with the right balance of nutrients.

The advantages of a Mediterranean diet include:

• Reducing Trans and saturated fat. But only in moderation, is saturated fat necessary. Your LDL (bad) cholesterol may rise if you consume too much-saturated fat. If your LDL level is high, you have a higher risk of forming arterial plaque (atherosclerosis). Your health will suffer if you consume trans-fat.

• Encourages the consumption of good unsaturated fats like omega-3 fatty acids, which are two of the "unhealthy fats" that can cause inflammation. Unsaturated fats promote healthy cholesterol levels, reduce inflammation, and improve brain health. A diet high in unsaturated fats and low in saturated fat also supports maintaining healthy blood sugar levels.

It restricts sodium. You run a higher risk of having a heart attack or stroke if you consume a lot of sodium in your diet.

• Regulates processed carbs, such as sugar, to a minimum. Your blood sugar may surge if you consume a lot of processed food. Furthermore, refined carbs are high in calories but low in nutritional value. These meals frequently contain little to no fiber, for instance.

• Preference for foods rich in fiber and antioxidants. Your body's inflammation can be decreased with the use of these nutrients. Additionally, fiber keeps the large intestine's capacity for waste absorption open. By preventing free radicals, antioxidants help you from developing cancer.

How does the Mediterranean diet appear?

Everybody's version of the Mediterranean diet is different. Generally speaking, it contains substantial amounts of whole grains, vegetables, and fruit, as well as a reasonable amount of fish, legumes, and nuts. Some serving guidelines and advice that dietitians frequently suggest are included in the chart below. It's crucial to discuss your unique needs and goals with a dietitian so you can create a strategy that works for you.

Mediterranean Diet Health Benefits

The Mediterranean diet is well-known for its purportedly beneficial effects on health because of its high intake of produce.

Three to nine servings of vegetables and up to two servings of fruit are commonly consumed each day by those following a Mediterranean diet.

Since they contain a variety of disease-preventing antioxidants, people who eat a diet rich in these fresh, whole foods have a lower risk of contracting an illness. Whether these advantages are brought about by antioxidants, other substances, or simply by having healthy eating habits generally, scientists are unaware of the precise reason for these advantages.

These potential health benefits of the Mediterranean diet are listed below.

Enhanced Heart Health

The advantage of this food plan for heart health may be its best-known trait. It reduces mortality from cardiovascular diseases and, in part, lowers cholesterol levels, which lowers the risk of heart disease.

A Lower Risk of Certain Cancers

Similarly to this, the Mediterranean diet has been linked to a lower risk of acquiring several head and neck cancers, colon cancer, prostate cancer, and breast cancer.

Lower Risk of Depression and a Sunnier Mood

You'll feel better physically, but your mental health will also improve if eating the Mediterranean way encourages you to eat more fruit and vegetables. According to research, people who consume more raw produce—especially dark leafy greens like spinach, fresh berries, and cucumbers—are less likely to have depressive symptoms and report feeling happier and more satisfied with their lives.

A Mediterranean eating pattern may help to improve mental health and lessen the symptoms of depression.

Decreased risk of neurodegenerative diseases

Studies have shown a correlation between consuming a Mediterranean-style diet and having better scores in general cognitive performance. The eating plan may slow down the aging process of the brain and reduce the risk of developing Alzheimer's and other types of dementia.

Lower risk of developing type 2diabetes and better diabetes management

A growing body of research indicates that maintaining a nutritious diet can help people with type 2 diabetes or those who are at risk for the disease stay healthy. First off, a review of the studies reveals that adopting a

Mediterranean diet enhances blood sugar regulation in persons who already have diabetes, indicating that it may be a helpful method to treat the condition. Additionally, adopting this diet can reportedly help people with diabetes improve their heart health because they are more likely to develop cardiovascular disease than people without the condition.

Decrease in complications from osteoarthritis

The Mediterranean diet may reduce the risk of disability, bone fractures, and weight gain (which can place additional pressure on the joints) because of its anti-inflammatory properties.

Find out more about the advantages of the Mediterranean diet for health.

Chapter three

Is weight loss possible with the Mediterranean diet?

The Mediterranean diet wasn't developed for weight loss; rather, it is a common way of eating in many civilizations around the world. One of the healthiest diets in the world also helps you maintain a healthy weight, as a matter of coincidence.

In one analysis of five trials including overweight and obese individuals, it was discovered that those who followed a Mediterranean diet lost up to 11 pounds (lb) more weight after one year than low-fat eaters.

They lost a total of between 9 and 22 pounds and kept it off for a year. However, the same study also discovered that other diets, such as the American Diabetes Association diet and low-carb diets, caused equal weight loss. The outcomes point to the fact that "there is no perfect diet for achieving sustained weight loss in overweight or obese adults," according to the researchers.

Although it avoids gimmicks and doesn't require calorie or macronutrient counting the way other diets (looking at you, ketogenic diet) do, a Mediterranean diet can be a varied and inclusive way to lose weight. It is filling as well, with an emphasis on good fats. Despite this, U.S. News & World Report ranked the Mediterranean diet No. 1 in 2022 in the category of "best diets overall" and No. 12 on its list of "best weight-loss diets."

It depends on your eating habits, according to researchers, who point out that it is not a given. The amount of fat consumed and the quantity of portions matter, even in a healthy diet like the Mediterranean.

Grocery list

Shopping at the store's outer edges, where the whole foods are often located, is always a good idea.

Choose foods that are high in nutrients whenever possible, such as fruits, vegetables, nuts, seeds, legumes, and whole grains.

A few staples for the Mediterranean diet are listed below for your shopping list:

• Vegetables: zucchini, mushrooms, broccoli, spinach, kale, onions, garlic, and carrots

• Frozen Vegetables: peas, carrots, broccoli, and mixed vegetables

Fruits and vegetables include apples, bananas, oranges, grapes, melons, peaches, pears, strawberries, and blueberries. Grains include quinoa, brown rice, oats, and whole-grain pasta. Tubers include potatoes, sweet potatoes, and yams.

• Legumes: kidney beans, black beans, chickpeas, and lentils

• Nuts, such as macadamia, cashew, walnut, pistachio, and almonds

Sunflower, pumpkin, chia, and hemp seeds are among the available seeds.

• Seasonings: oregano, cinnamon, cayenne pepper, sea salt, pepper, and pepper.

• Seafood items include salmon, sardines, mackerel, trout, shrimp, and mussels.

• Milk, Greek yogurt, and other dairy products

Eggs include chicken, quail, and duck eggs in addition to poultry (chicken, duck, and turkey).

Extra virgin olive oil, olives, avocados, and avocado oil are examples of healthy fats.

An extensive list of foods to eat on the Mediterranean diet

On the Mediterranean diet, the following foods will make up a sizable portion of your diet, whereas processed foods will be strictly prohibited. Processed foods include prepared sweets like cookies, cake, and chocolates as well as salty packaged snacks like potato chips and crackers. Other examples of processed foods include cold cuts, sausage, and other processed meats.

You can choose to indulge with some dark chocolate and red wine. The nutritional information for the following foods is given for your convenience, even though the Mediterranean diet does not require you to count calories.

Almond Oil

119 calories, 0 grams of protein, 13.5 grams of fat, 2 grams of saturated fat, 10 grams of monounsaturated fat, 0 grams of carbohydrates, 0 grams of fiber, and 0 grams of sugar are contained in each tablespoon.

Benefits: Research suggests that switching from foods heavy in saturated fats (like butter) to sources of monounsaturated fatty acids from plants, such as olive oil, can reduce the risk of heart disease by 19%.

Tomatoes

32 calories, 1.6 grams of protein, 0 grams of fat, 7 grams of carbs, 2 grams of fiber, and 5 grams of sugar are contained in one serving of one cup (chopped).

The benefits they contain include lycopene, an antioxidant with potent anti-carcinogenic properties linked to a lower risk of various cancers, including breast and prostate cancer. To guard against cardiovascular disease, additional tomato ingredients may help lower the risk of blood clots.

Salmon

130 calories, 21 grams of protein, 4.5 grams of fat, 0 grams of carbs, and 0 grams of fiber are contained in 1 small fillet.

Benefits One of the main sources of omega-3 fatty acids is fatty fish. Eat at least two fish meals each week, preferably fatty fish like salmon, for a healthy heart.

Walnuts

Per 1 ounce (14 halves) serving 185 calories, 4 grams of protein, 18.5 grams of fat, 2 grams of saturated fat, 3 grams of monounsaturated fat, 13 grams of polyunsaturated fat, 4 grams of carbohydrate, 2 grams of fiber, and 1 gram of sugar

Benefits A tiny study involving 18 healthy individuals found that these nuts, which are high in heart-protective polyunsaturated fats, may also have positive effects on your gut microbiota (and hence enhance digestive health), as well as lower LDL cholesterol.

Chickpeas

Benefits per serving of 1 cup: 210 calories, 11 grams of protein, 4 grams of fat, 35 grams of carbohydratcs, and 10 grams of fiber. Chickpeas, the primary component of hummus, are a good source of fiber; they provide iron, zinc, folate, and magnesium, as well as benefits for weight loss and intestinal health.

Arugula

5 calories, 0.5 grams of protein, 0 grams of fat, 1 gram of carbohydrate, 0 grams of fiber, and 0 grams of sugar are contained in 1 cup of the food.

Benefits Under this way of eating, leafy greens like arugula are consumed in large quantities. A study found that eating leafy greens frequently (more than six times per week) as part of a Mediterranean-style diet decreased the risk of Alzheimer's disease.

Pomegranate

Every half-cup serving (arils) has 72 calories, 1.5 g protein, 1 g fat, 16 g carbs, 4 g fiber, and 12 g sugar

Benefits In all its vivid crimson splendor, this fruit is packed with potent polyphenols that fight inflammation and free radicals. According to a study, it has been hypothesized that pomegranates also possess anticancer effects.

Lentils

116 calories, 9 grams of protein, 0 grams of fat, 20 grams of carbohydrates, 8 grams of fiber, and 2 grams of sugar per serving of 1/2 cup.

Benefits According to research, replacing half of your portion of a high-glycemic carbohydrate (such as rice) with lentils reduces the glycemic response by 20%.

Ferro contains 190 calories, 6g of protein, 1g of fat, 38 g of carbohydrates, 5g of fiber, and 0g of sugar per 14 cups (uncooked) serving.

Benefits Ferro and other whole grains are the foundation of this diet. Exceptionally satisfying protein and fiber are offered by this grain. Consuming whole grains has been associated with a lower risk of several diseases, such as type 2 diabetes, colon cancer, heart disease, and stroke.

Greek yogurt

20 grams of protein, 8 grams of carbs, no fiber, 7 grams of sugar, 2 grams of saturated fat, 1 gram of monounsaturated fat, and 4 grams of total fat are all contained in each 7-ounce container of the low-fat plain.

Benefits Dairy products are an excellent source of calcium, even when they are consumed in moderation. You can cut back on your consumption of saturated fat by choosing low- or no-fat options.

Chapter four

How to Eat Out While Following the Mediterranean Diet: Guidelines

Visiting a restaurant? You might follow the Mediterranean diet and be satisfied if you use these tips.

1. Place a high premium on vegetables.

Vegetables are heavily emphasized in the Mediterranean diet, so look for dishes that are loaded with them. These are typically available in the salad, side, and appetizer sections of the menu. As an alternative, start your dinner with roasted vegetables or a salad.

Ask them to leave out the condiments and drizzle some extra virgin olive oil on top.

2. Choose the Fish

If you enjoy fish but find it challenging to eat it frequently at home, ask for it when you're out at a restaurant, and the chef will prepare it specifically for you. If you frequently order red meat when eating out, this could have a big influence. Consider choosing fatty seafood that is high in omega-3 fatty acids.

Even though tuna and mackerel may occasionally appear on the menu, salmon is generally available and simple to locate.

3. Keep Alcohol to a Minimum

If you use alcohol, choose a glass of red wine occasionally rather than a margarita or a beer, which you can sip while eating. Occasionally, stick to sparkling plain water with a lemon or lime wedge rather than drinking any alcohol at all.

4. Enjoy Fruit as a Dessert

Fresh fruit is typically eaten as dessert in a variety of cultures.

You can ask if they can bring you a tiny fruit cup to end your dinner, even though fresh fruit isn't typically on the dessert menu at restaurants. A plate of berries or a few slices of melons can be prepared at home if you decide to forgo dessert entirely.

Basic Mediterranean Diet Tips to Remember

The Mediterranean diet can be started and maintained with the assistance of a trained dietitian-nutritionist, which you can locate at Eatright.org. However, these suggestions might also be useful.

1. Be selective about the sources of fat you consume, and refrain from overindulging.

You can lower the amount of saturated fat in your diet by avoiding eating a lot of red or processed meat and relying more on foods high in monounsaturated fatty acids, such as avocado, almonds, and olive oil.

These fats don't result in higher cholesterol, contrary to what saturated fats do. As good sources of fat, Cohen recommends nut oils, fish oils, and olive oil. If you are careless, you might consume more fat than is advised for daily consumption, including healthy fat. According to the U.S. Department of Health and Human Services, you should aim to consume 20 percent to 35 percent of your daily calories as fat, with saturated fats making up no more than 10 percent of your total calorie consumption.

2. Take adequate calcium supplements.

The Mediterranean diet is permissible, but only in moderation when it comes to calcium-rich foods like cheese and yogurt. In addition to kale, sardines, and other non-dairy foods like fortified almond milk, Cohen suggests looking for calcium-enriched versions of these foods.

3. Set aside a time in your schedule to prepare meals.

Even if you don't have to spend all day in the kitchen, you still need to cook because the diet revolves around using wholesome, delicious fresh foods. You can experience a learning curve as you develop these abilities.

4. Modify Your Favorite Recipes to Be Compatible with the Mediterranean Diet

This diet makes meal preparation simple because there is such a wide selection of complete, fresh foods available. Additionally, you don't have to get rid of your favorites; they might just need some adjustments. For instance, you might select a pizza with a lot of vegetables instead of one with sausage and pepperoni. Additionally, you can eat a variety of items in one sitting. By filling up fresh fruit and vegetables, you can increase the volume of your meals while consuming fewer calories.

Don't drink too much or too often.

Along with the consumption of red wine in moderation, one of the traits that set the Mediterranean diet apart is the fact that it is seen as being so healthy. Women should only have one glass, while men should continue to have no more than two. If breast cancer runs in your family, drinking any alcohol raises your risk of getting the disease.

Consult your doctor to determine the best course of action for you in this case.

Summary

Dietary Guidelines for Maintaining Health

Both Mediterranean and macrobiotic diets are very effective at preventing heart disease, obesity, and chronic diseases due to the large portions of nutrient-dense vegetables, fruits, nuts, seeds, and grains that they both contain. Contrarily, the Mediterranean diet does not emphasize specific serving sizes. It might be difficult for those trying to lose weight since they are unclear about how much of each category you should eat.

According to the Strengthening Health version, 25% of the macrobiotic diet must consist of grains, 25% of legumes, 25% of vegetables, and 25% of fruit, nuts, and seeds. Utilizing these fundamental recommendations, people will find it simpler to determine how much food they should consume and what meals to make.

The inability to lose weight and keep it off is a problem that diets frequently face. In addition to having food addictions and desires for processed foods, we might also eat out of emotion. 38 percent of adults claim to have overindulged or consumed unhealthily in the previous month due to stress.

After overindulging in extremely unhealthy meals, more than one-third of people (36%) say they feel drowsy or sleepy, and half of the adults (49%) say they feel dissatisfied with themselves as a result. Additionally, 46% of people say they feel awful about their physical appearance. The Mediterranean diet does not emphasize the more challenging aspects of adhering to a diet, even while it promotes spending time with family and being physically active. The macrobiotic diet was developed to identify meals that improve one's sense of self and physical well-being. It is based on ancient civilizations.

Both the macrobiotic diet practice and the Mediterranean diet have many advantages, but the macrobiotic diet practice is more effective when it comes to helping you alter your life. For starters, have a look at a few quick and easy macrobiotic recipes. The macrobiotic diet instructs us to become conscious of our pressures, seek out meals that support our mental and physical development, and forge a bond with the cosmos. Find out more about the macrobiotic courses we offer.

www.ingramcontent.com/pod-product-compliance
Lightning Source LLC
LaVergne TN
LVHW020536160826
845677LV00015B/4084

* 9 7 9 8 3 7 0 5 4 9 0 5 2 *